MASTERING THE ART OF GREAT LENGTHS

Jessica Ivette Gonzalez

AuthorHouse™
1663 Liberty Drive
Bloomington, IN 47403
www.authorhouse.com
Phone: 1 (800) 839-8640

Published by AuthorHouse 09/05/2018

ISBN: 978-1-5462-5582-6 (sc)
ISBN: 978-1-5462-5583-3 (e)

Library of Congress Control Number: 2018909802

Print information available on the last page.

author house

LASH ARTISTRY
STUDENT TRAINING MANUAL

Author
Jessica Ivette Gonzalez

Welcome to the exciting career of lash artistry. In a fast growing industry with an abundant number of product distribution companies worldwide, this particular curriculum is designed to empower, educate, and fuel fire of wisdom in you as the next certified lash specialist.

The highly extensive curriculum provides a wealth of information to provide clarity, structure and a path for *all* beginners as well as seasoned artist who want to brush up on their skills. Lash Artistry is no longer just an additional service to add on to your professional resume; but a massive game changer in your career.

In this explosive career move so many questions arise! Which product is the best? Which company offers the best training? Why should you offer this service? These are just a few questions running around in your creative mind. The training at Lash Esthetica and its affiliates aim is to share the wealth of knowledge from experience for over 12 years and beyond. The mission is to instill a passion and integrity for the industry as a whole.

Welcome to your journey as a future lash specialist.

I Love Lashing With Passion...I wish the same for you!

Jessica Gonzalez

Contents

CHAPTER ONE

EYELASH EXTENSIONS BASICS

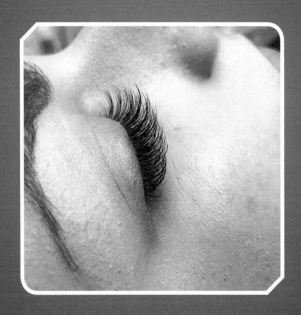

"ALWAYS STRIVE TO BE BETTER THAN YESTERDAY"

JESSICA GONZALEZ

THE BASICS OF SYNTHETIC EYELASH EXTENSIONS

A synthetic lash extension is the most common type of extension. Synthetic is a type of plastic extension that can be *firm, stiff* or *lighter*, and vary in *flexibility*. Materials common for lash fibers can be silk, sable or synthetic (plastic). The most common used is MINK (which falls under synthetic). There are several hundred manufacturers and distributors in the market in high demand offering quality products in the lash industry. Be creative. Explore as many products to determine for yourself what works best for your taste and environment (state, climate, treatment room, humidity factors); your consumer niche, and the selection you would like to offer your clients.

LENGTH & DIAMETER

Extensions come in various sizes ranging generally from a 6mm-17mm in length. (Short to long) The diameters that are the most common for classic individual extensions are: 0.15, 0.18, 0.2 and 0.25.

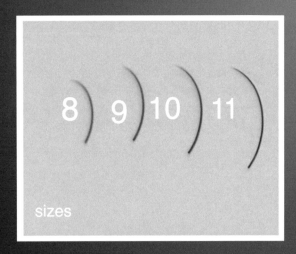

sizes

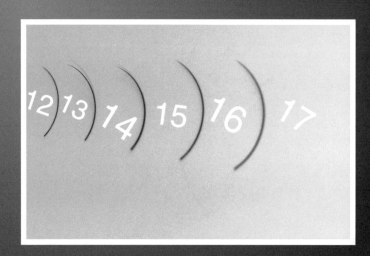

Sizing on a client should be determined based on the natural hair structure. Be realistic on the decision to determine if the hair is strong enough to hold the chosen lash. Observe the integrity of the hair, determine the cycle of the current hair stage and compare it to the neighboring natural lash lengths to best determine the hair growth and stage for the appropriate length and diameter extension.

The thickness discussed below is for the traditional classic application of individual one on one application of an (1) extension to a (1) natural lash. Doubling up lash extensions on 1 natural hair will cause damage to the natural hair. Advance techniques will be discussed later in your course.

Deciding on the appropriate diameter for your client
The diameters I discuss here are the most common in the industry. But there are many more. The following is a basic introduction to diameters and a guide on what you feel is best for you.

0.15 is the thinnest in *classic* application technique. It is important to know that many thinner diameters are available, but reserved for use in advance techniques for hybrid and volume lashing. Usually the appearance of depth is difficult to achieve for a 1 on 1 application of an extension. This diameter is recommended for the client who has experienced discomfort due to sensitive lids; or shows signs of irritant symptoms, but can still wear lash extensions. *It's important to maximize on every natural lash possible during application.

0.18 is a diameter that is gaining popularity now versus the 0.2. I highly advise not going thicker in diameter of lashes beyond the 0.18. This is an ideal diameter that allows a fuller look, minimizes surrounding natural lashes during application to bond to the extension so easily; therefore allows the separation technique to be performed with less discomfort to the client.

0.2 is the most popular thickness allowing for depth, and volume while not weighing down the natural lash.

0.25 is stiffest and thicker. Recommended *NOT* to be used on everyone. Being selective. A coarse hair typically can hold this diameter creating a dense look. This particular diameter can be heavy for the natural lash and feel stiff. Does not allow for easy movement of the natural lash.

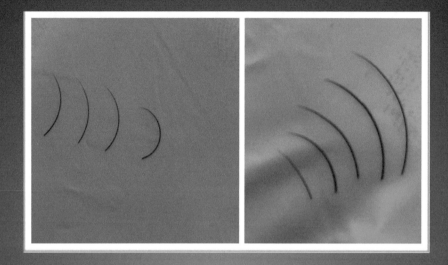

Shapes comparison: (L) image: ex. B, N, C, D I Size comparison: (R) image: ex. 6,8,10, 14

CURL STRUCTURE (SHAPE)

The general shapes are *B, N or J, C, CC, D Curl.* The options are endless when it comes to creating a look. Usually, the natural lash curl will provide a clue for the best shape to use. In addition to the natural lash, other facial factors play a role to achieve the overall desired look for your client. The "Face Factors" will be discussed in page 48 in Chapter 5 " EMPOWERING & CUSTOMIZE ". Options are available for the unique shape of the natural lash.

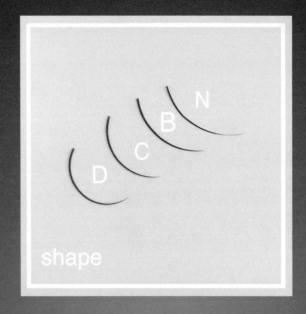

shape

B Curl - perfect for a straight lash that directs downward. B Shape is designed to plane the downward growing lash up away from the eye. The suspension of weight at the base of the B lash pulls the clients natural lash to lift up unlike the N/J curl. *Attachment 100% of the natural lash.*

N or J Curl- similar to shape of a normal lash. Straight out and a little lift. No suspension to the natural lash. *Attachment 100% of the natural lash.*

C Curl- A perfect curl that compliments most faces. Ideal for the client who uses a lash curler tool during the application of mascara. *Attachment 80-100% of the natural lash.*

D Curl- for the natural lash that is super short or has a perm like lash. The D has a curl that grabs the natural short lash and supports the curl. It grabs the most kinky shaped lash that has it's own attitude. *Attachment will be 20%-35% of the natural lash.*

Hint: Stock up on the *B curl* and *C curl.* The B shape is designed to directly plane the natural lash in an upward direction from the base lifting away from the eye. The B Shape is an alternative to the N/J shape because the curl appears to have a greater lift. C shape is a great curl also for general use. The D shape is a good curl to have for clients with short lashes, of different ethnic backgrounds, or due to health issues causing hair loss to be significant. Grow your client foundation and after much observation, then determine if the inventory is worth carrying.

The house without a foundation…

Building a house is serious business. A proper foundation of the house is important for the success of the final build out. Without the framework, a house cannot be built. Ok, so your full set of extensions isn't a house but failing to have a selection of sizes will create unbalanced symmetry and irregular shedding in between lash fills. You must learn the importance of curls and sizes. Selection of a minimum of 3 sizes is the foundation of your work. Long glamorous lashes look magical for a few days then not so much. It's important to think about how the lashes will look 2-3 weeks later. You want the mileage on those lashes. Do you want to find yourself doing full sets every 2-3 weeks? Or fills? Improper selection of lashes look unattractive and lead to discomfort around the delicate eye area.

The size of the extension and diameter applied to the lash adds to the weight. Incorrect sizing can cause the natural lash to shed prematurely. When this happens, the client can suffer from a condition called *TRACTION ALOPECIA.*

* Traction Alopecia - Reference in Pathology section of this manual.

COLORS

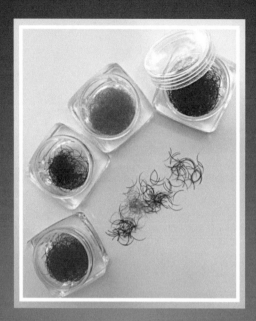

Black is the traditional choice to replace the desire to use mascara. A selection of a rainbow of colors gives a twist of fun. From the conservative to the outlandish consumer, be bold and have fun playing with lashes! Brown works great for the timid attitude... yet purple fires up brown eyes. Blue maximizes the natural color of the client with blue/gray hues in the iris; green gives the eye a pop! Yet pink, outrageous and fabulous!

Would lashes in different colors be in demand for your demographics?

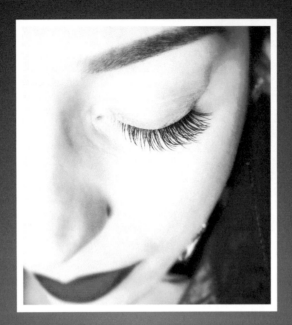

The hype about MINK

When ordering Mink lashes from a distributor or a direct manufacturer, the product will have slight differences in the shape, thickness in diameter, feel, and in shine or gloss appearance. *IMPORTANT TO KNOW

For example: You purchase a mink brand from company (1) and company (2). Exact size and diameter; but you may notice that it looks slightly different. This is common and to be expected. In general, mink should feel softer than a traditional synthetic lash with more bend and flexibility. It should diminish or limit the poking against the lid from the blinking action of the eye. Mink selections do vary from company to company. Search for the one you personally like more.

Synthetic lashes generally are stiffer, more structured and less bend than the minx. Same concept applies to synthetic depending on the brand of choice.

*Please note the misconception that mink is animal material. Mink should be reference as a cut structure that allows bend and flexibility of synthetic material.

CHAPTER TWO

ANATOMY & PHYSIOLOGY

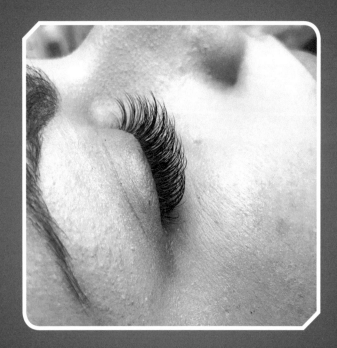

ANATOMY & PHYSIOLOGY OF THE EYE AREA

The information of the following is basic textbook information. Learning about the eye area structure helps to understand the sensitivity of the eye and why being graceful with your *mobility of hand placements* are important when you provide the service to your client. The knowledge of informing yourself with the basics of the eye and its general accessory structure is arming you with the understanding why it is important to practice a safe standard of application from start to finish. The smallest irritation to the eye area can cause an irritation that appears intimidating for a new artist; along with cause of alert on the client's perspective if not handled properly. During the time of your training you will gain a better understanding why... later in the chapter of pathology.

THE EYE STRUCTURE

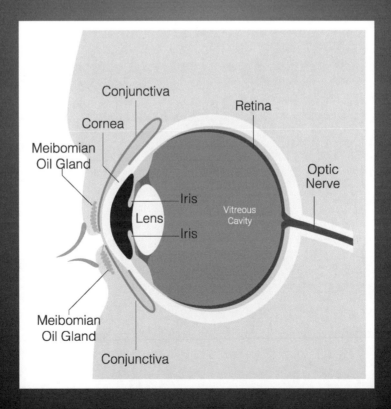

Important parts of the eyeball structure

1. RETINA is a basic nerve layer- lining the anterior portion of the eye. The function is to sense light along which creates impulses that travel through the optic nerve and communicates with the brain.
2. MACULA is the smallest area in the retina that houses special cells that are light sensitive. The macula is important in allowing the visual recognition of fine details and sees them clearly.
3. OPTIC NERVE is the nerve that connects between the attachments of the eye to the brain. The impulses created/formed by the retina is carried by the optic nerve. This particular nerve interprets the impulses into images for the brain to understand.
4. SCLERA is the white outer covering of the eyeball. The texture is thick and tough. The Conjunctiva is the moist mucous membrane that coats inner and outer surface of the eyelids. *Front of the eye only.*
5. VITREOUS is a jelly substance that is transparent in color and fills the center of the eye giving shape to the eyeball. The covering is connected to the pupil.
6. CORNEA serves as a filter, screening out damaging ultraviolet rays from the sunlight.
7. LENS is transparent inside of the eye, which focuses light rays onto the retina.

The fat surrounding the eye helps cushion the eye offering protection from the hard bone of the eye socket. The human eye is asymmetrical having slightly different measurements from the other. The orbital cavity (located in the skull where the eyes are attached) are supported by ligaments, muscles, and facial attachments/expansions around it. The extra ocular muscle allows the "orbit" movement of the eyeball. The extra ocular muscles allow the movement from side to side. The location of where the optic nerve leaves the retina is known as the blind spot. There are no photoreceptor cells in the blind spot. The tiny blood vessels in the eyes transport blood to the retina.

CELLS THAT DETERMINE COLOR PERCEPTION IN VISION

Rod Cells are the light sensors that are responsible for detecting colors such as black, white, and various shades of grey. These cells are integral for our night vision. The rod cells are used in peripheral vision and less intense light activates its use. There are an estimate 120 million cell sensors in the eye structure.

Cone cells function is to detect color and functions best in bright lighting and perception of fine details in the images. There are 7 million light sensors and 3 types of cells. Each cell is sensitive to one of the primary colors of red, blue and green.

The cone cells are located in the macula. In the brightest light, these cells are designed to provide an imagery that is clear, sharp and detect with use of color fine details. The rod cells are found in the outside of the macula and extend to the outer edge of the retina. The function is peripheral or side vision. Detection of motion is another function in the eye to see in dim light or allows vision during the night, i.e., driving.

EYELID

The eyelid is the covering of the human eye that provides protection. The main function of the eyelid is protection of the corneal, for the nutrition of the corneal, and spreads the tears and other secretions of the eye surface. The client's natural lashes provide additional protection from foreign objects and particles from entering the eye and causing injury to the eye. As mentioned earlier, the skin in the eye area is the thinnest in the inner lid towards the nose and gradually thickening towards the outer upper lid corner. The lower lid also is the same in skin thinness.

TEARS

The tears produced provide a lubrication that keeps your eyes healthy and protect them from irritants. There are several types of tears comprised of *water, fats, sugars, and proteins.* I will address the most important ones that can occur during the service.

One of the fluids of tears most common is the *Basel Tears (BT), which* is present in the eye that keeps the cornea moist and nourished. Because the cornea has no blood vessels or supply of blood flow, it depends on this tear secretion for its oxygen supply that comes from air. The Basel tear also creates an even smooth layer for optical quality. Every time you blink, it reforms, and reduces bacteria that adheres to the surface of the eye. Proteins plays a role as the antibiotic to kill off the bacteria. Another function of the BT is to reduce friction due to movement of the eye.

Reflex Tears is a second kind of secretion but is a result of sudden external stimulus; for example, a foreign object, such as dust or vapors in the air. The reflex tear purpose is to immediately wash out irritants that come in contact with the eye.

In the inner portion towards the nasal area, the hair is finer. There is more sebaceous glands making it an area of tears of *oil secretion tears.*

The Lacrimal gland begins the production of tears that drains through small canals called canaliculus into the puncta; a small hole located in the upper and lower lid. The tears then travel and drains into the nasolcrimal duct to drain through the nose.

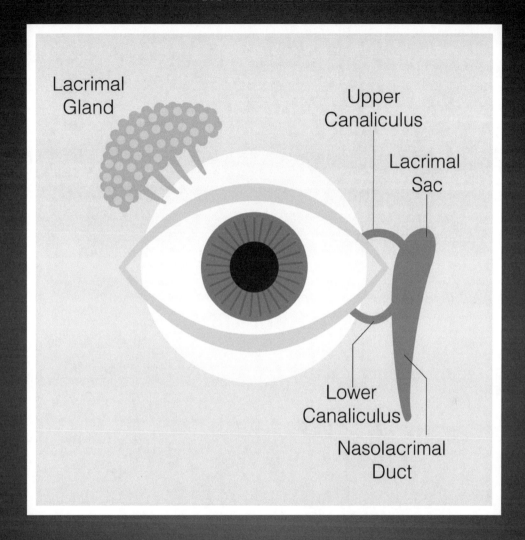

Lacrimal Gland

Upper Canaliculus

Lacrimal Sac

Lower Canaliculus

Nasolacrimal Duct

Tip: During the procedure the client may begin to tear. Use a cotton swab and gently place in the inner eye while closed to absorb the tears.

EYELASH GROWTH AND FUNCTION

The eyelash grows from the actual eyelid at the base of waterline. The purpose of the eyelash is a mechanical function similar to wipers on a car. It has a sweeping action that transports dirt, oil secretion, makeup, and environmental pollution debris preventing from getting inside the eye and prevents serious injury to the function of the eye. The eye area is vulnerable due to the epidermal layer of the skins thinness. It takes very little to irritate the area causing redness and inflammation.

The lash undergoes through 3 important cycles of growth leading to a 4th silent stage of shedding (when the lash finally detaches) making way for a new *Anagen* hair to extract from the opening of the eyelid. In this particular training, we will discuss more in detail the basic first 3 stages of eyelash growth as one of the most important topics to educate the client during the service, about aftercare, expectations of longevity of a set of lash extensions and future maintenance.

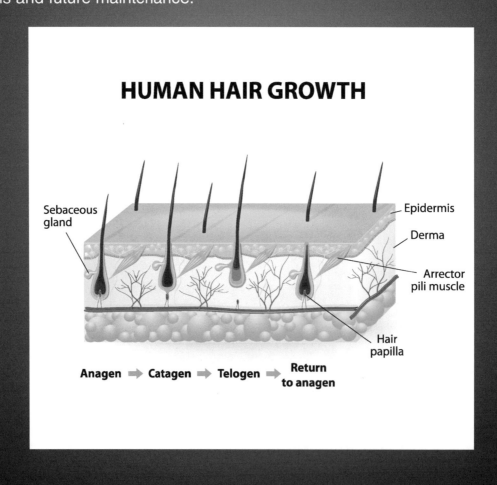

HAIR CYCLE

The hair has 3 stages of growth. Starting from the Anagen stage (baby), Catagen stage (teen), and Telogen stage (adult). For each client, the length of lashes will vary and also the natural thickness. The natural lash grows to an estimated 10mm in length varying client to client. Everyone is unique. The average growth cycle estimation is 30-60 days. The Anagen stage typically will require a 6-10mm extension. Catagen is 8,10,12, and Telogen usually can hold a 10, 12, and a 14mm extension. This is only a suggested sizing as each client is unique. In depth more details will be discussed further in the Chapter "The Art of Framing". Diligent training leads to confidence on selecting which lash extension is appropriate for the natural hair.

Of course, in the lash industry long millimeter lashes are available starting at size 15 and up. Use discretion and common sense if you plan to provide such sizes. Ask yourself "Can the natural hair of the client support the length?" The integrity of the natural lash with respect to the growth stages is vital for the health of the natural lash. Note: when the last stage of the natural lash completes the cycle the average internal portion of the lash (internal part in the eyelid during the Telogen stage) is estimated 1-2 millimeters supporting the external portion of the lash (portion of the natural lash exposed from the lid). The base of the natural lash job is to provide support. The extension should not compromise the integrity of the natural lash.

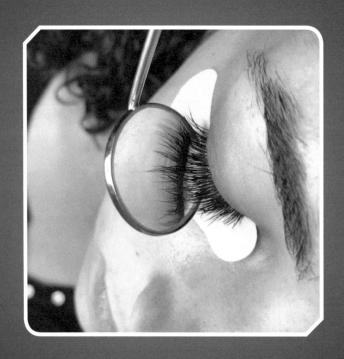

CHAPTER THREE

PATHOLOGY

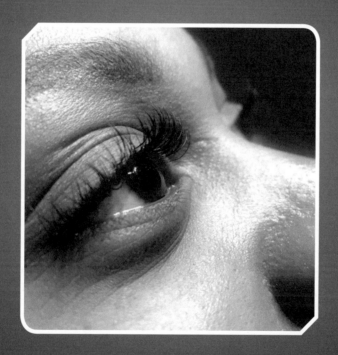

"LASH WITH PASSION"

PATHOLOGY

The eyelash extension industry has completed a decade of gathering valuable information such as: understanding the retention obstacles, training efficiency, products and tools; but most importantly, having a better understanding of pathology.

Each client is chemically and physically unique. Factors of internal and external factors play a role. It is important to have a general understanding of different experiences that can arise with each client. Understanding the body's internal environment combined with external physical environment will help you handle uncomfortable situations, determine the possible causes and resolve the matter with confidence.

The health of the client does play a role in the experience he/she will have from the start of the service and in the long run. Several eye disorders/disease will be discussed along with other contraindications. Basic knowledge will help you to access the awareness of an allergic reaction versus an irritant that can be possibly prevented. Other disorders of the body will determine if the client is a good or bad candidate for eyelash extensions. Remember, you are not a doctor or a medical advisor. Diagnosing is outside of your scope of practice as a lash specialist. Build a network of professional medical partners you can refer your client to.

Reactions will occur from time to time during your practice. Reactions can occur for a number of reasons. Not limited to adhesive, following are some contributors:

Tape, cleansers, primers, gel patches, eye stickers, and the lash extensions material. A client who has no previous issues can develop sensitivity or have a full-blown reaction after long term wear.

A reaction will involve swelling, itching but irritants are usually minor. It is important to document the irritant. It could occur that one time, but it also could be a starting indication that a potential reaction will occur in a future visit for a lash fill.

This chapter will discuss common ocular disorders in the area of eye disease.

COMMON OCULAR DISORDERS
Blepharitis

Blepharitis is the inflammation of the eyelash follicles. The visual effect will be directly on the eyelid. Some clients will have Blepharitis due to other factors but allergic Blepharitis does happen with lash extensions, and you should be informed.

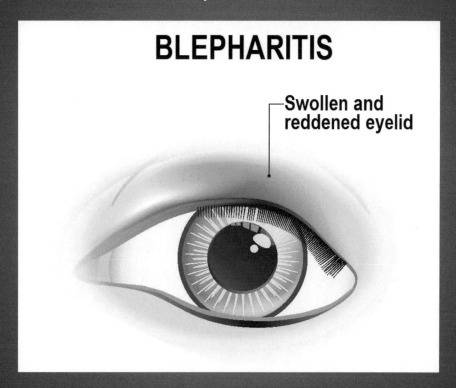

BLEPHARITIS

Swollen and reddened eyelid

Symptoms:

Swelling, redness/pink, itching, crust buildup, flaking skin, dry skin that will peel, dandruff of the eye. Though there are different causes for Blepharitis below are 3 different types to be familiar with: *Bacterial, Seborrheic, and Gland dysfunction.*

- **Bacterial** Blepharitis is an eye infection that is very common. Staphylococcus bacteria, which is common on skin (the nostrils also; which is close to the eye area). Imagine scratching an area of your skin then rubbing your eyes. Wash hands regularly. However the problem with bacteria is when there is overgrowth the infection begins and parts of or the whole eye begins to show signs. It can be an acute onset or a chronic uncomfortable problem. The client should be provided appropriate aftercare instructions and products after the lash service for home use. The client must understand the importance of regular good eye hygiene care. It is essential.

- **Seborrheic** Blepharitis is typically caused by allergies or triggered by an irritant in physical or chemical substances found in our environment. For example; detergents, cosmetics, dust particles in the air, extreme change in temperature and humidity. Also commonly known as eczema or psoriasis in the eye area.

- **Meibomian Gland Dysfunction** is the leading cause of dry eye. The meibomian glands are found in the lid top and bottom. There are an estimate 20-40 glands on both upper and lower lid. The glands function is to secret oil slowing the evaporation of our tears we produce. The abnormality or dysfunction of the glands leads to dry eye syndrome and associated with Blepharitis. A person who wears contacts on a regular bases not allowing rest and oxygen to circulate in between use can lead to dry eye syndrome and potential other eye health issues.

CONJUNCTIVITIS (commonly called "pink eye")

An infection or swelling in the outer membrane of the protective layer of the "front" of the eye. Blood vessels within the membrane become inflamed. The inflamed mucous membrane (covers the eye called conjunctiva) becomes a bright rich red or pink color. Usually affecting one eye or both.

Types of conjunctivitis

Allergic conjunctivitis

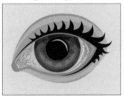

- there is itching and redness of the eye, swelling of the conjunctiva and the eyelid

Viral conjunctivitis

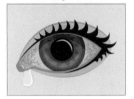

- redness of the eyes and periodic itching, increased lacrimation

Bacterial conjunctivitis

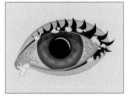

- redness, dryness of the eyes and the skin around them, mucopurulent discharge

Common symptoms*you are not able to diagnose outside of your scope of practice; always refer your client to seek medical attention when appropriate.*
- Red/ Pink conjunctiva
- Gritty feeling (having small particles/ sand like)
- A discharge consistency of watery to a thick fluid that builds up around the eye. Occurring during the night.
- Eyes can feel sealed together.
- Itchiness
- Abnormal amount of tear production

What causes conjunctivitis?

Allergies - allergens to external environment. Pollen is the example that can irritate the eye and stimulates the body to create more histamines, causing inflammation to trigger a response to what it is communicated as an infection. An allergic trigger is usually itchy.

Doctor usually prescribe an antihistamine to stop the inflammation.
Over the counter medications commonly available: Claritin (Loratadine), and Benadryl (diphenhydramine), as well as other treatment antihistamine or anti-inflammatory eye drops. Refer your client to a doctor for recommendations.

Chemicals from a foreign substance or chemical agents spritz into the eye. For example, chlorine common in swimming pools can cause conjunctivitis. When an irritation from a foreign substance comes into contact with the eye, flush with water, which can be effective in preventing the chemical irritant from pink eye to come into full bloom.

Bacteria is a common and spreads easily especially among young children. Keeping your workstation and tools sanitized and clean will help the spread of bacteria in the working environment and keep your staff, clients, and you safe. Medical attention would be advised for proper ointments and antibiotic medication recommendations. Will usually go away in just a few days.

Shared cosmetics are a common factor for eye infections.
Other factors - Improper fitting contacts or decorative contacts

Virus has no treatment. It is much like catching the common cold. No cures for a virus. The symptoms usually go away on its own within 7-10 days, after the virus has run its course of action. Helpful suggestions: warm compress of water will help calm and soothe your symptoms.

FOREIGN OBJECTS

Foreign particle enters the eye from the external environment such a dust or a metal shard. This can cause not just discomfort but pain. Immediately affects the cornea and or the conjunctiva.

The cornea is a clear dome that covers the front surface of the eye. It serves as a protective covering for the front of the eye. Light enters the eye through the cornea. It also helps focus light on the retina at the back of the eye.

Common symptoms

- Pressure or discomfort
- Sensation of an object in your eye
- Eye pain
- More than light sensitivity - borderline pain
- Excessive blinking
- Redness / bloodshot eye
- Extreme tearing (streaming tears)
- Can have discharge or blood in the eye. Uncommon for a lash artist to have a client in this situation.

Common *intraocular objects* (foreign object that penetrates into the eye)

- Natural eyelashes (when an eyelash extension gets in the eye, it's painful!)
- Dried mucus
- Sawdust
- Dirt
- Sand
- Cosmetics
- Contact lenses
- Metal particles
- Glass shards

When fragments enter the eye, it is usually caused by wind or falling debris in the atmosphere. More severe cases such as from an accident have a high risk of injury with long-term consequences. In the lash industry, not so much risk...but risk is still present in general no matter how minor.

DRY EYE SYNDROME

The eye does not produce enough tears to effectively keep your eyes moist. Tears help /aid in keeping enough moisture in your eyes. The syndrome is very common. The symptoms can be stinging / burning and extremely uncomfortable. For example straining the eye / sever focusing can cause dry eye. There are over the counter solutions for dry eye. A lash extension that is thinner in diameter (.15m) will be a wiser choice to avoid potential discomfort. The eyelid in the crease of the upper and lower lid of the outer eye can become irritated so avoiding extensions in the outer corners can also aid in comfort for the client.

Tears are a mixture of water, oils, and mucus. An imbalance can cause dry eye. If for example the *meibomian* glands are clogged, the oily part of the tears slows down evaporation -> *low quality tears.*

Common causes for dry eye
- Deficiency of vitamin A
- Diabetes, lupus, rheumatoid arthritis, allergies, infections, and thyroid disorders.
- Chemical burns (some gel patches in the market can cause a chemical burn to the eye depending on the ingredients in the gel substance)
- Damage to the tear gland from injury, inflammation
- Laser eye surgery (Lasik - usually a temporary side effect)

If left untreated can be painful, cause ulcers or scars on your cornea (the front part of the eye); decrease quality of performing everyday tasks that require focusing.

Treatment - Eye drops over the counter or prescription from a medical doctor.

CORNEAL ABRASIONS

Have you ever experienced a paper cut?

It stings tremendously and it feels like a grain of sand is floating around. Seek medical attention immediately. Chronic abrasions can create long-term effects without proper treatment.

The cornea contains many nerve endings. A minor scratch is very uncomfortable and painful. It feels like there is something large and rough in the eye. You search for it, but most of the time you can't see exactly the location. *In a case that a client experiences a corneal abrasion, advice them to seek medical attention immediately. A dislodged eyelash extension can cause a corneal abrasion. Client should avoid touching, rubbing any part of the eye. In most cases, an antibiotic is going to be the best solution to ease discomfort.

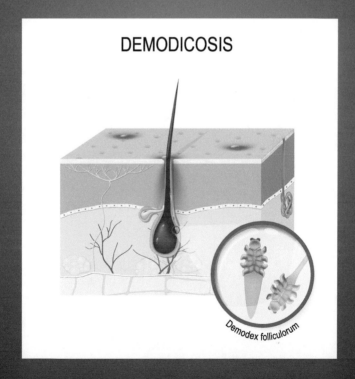

DEMODICOSIS

Demodex folliculorum

DEMODEX MITE

Microscopic creatures that live on the skin and hair but become a nuisance. This nasty mite lives inside of the eyelash, eyebrow and facial hair follicles not excluding the sebaceous glands associated with these hairs. Feeding on dead skin cells, hormones, and oil.

(Sebaceous secretion). The mite anchors by their scales feeding away. Proper hygiene is important especially after care protocol that only the client has control of. There are no symptoms as demodex is a natural body organism. When the mites over grow, it leads to *Blepharitis*. This can cause premature hair shedding and also effect the actual grow of the natural eyelash at the present time of the mite overgrowth. The mites take up the space preventing the natural hair cycle and in severe cases, lash loss can occur. A weak / compromised immune system can cause an over infestation or just plan lack of eyelid hygiene practices. Clients should remove all makeup and cleanser regularly. There are different makeup remover pads and cleaners to aid in cleaning the lash.

Provide your client with after care products for purchase or complimentary after the service. If your client has a demodex infestation, recommend seeking professional medical assistance.

CONTACT DERMATITIS
Reference to Blepharitis / Allergen

- The size and diameter of the lash extensions can irritate aggressively sensitive lids that have a general problem.
- Thick extensions can cause dermatitis. (.25) and on occasion (.2)
- When placed too close to the skin, rubbing, poking on the skin, dislodging, and improper placement can all be negative contributors to creating a problem that could have been prevented.
- The symptoms of an allergic reaction versus an irritant is much the same and hard to tell apart.

- *Physical trauma can cause Dermatitis...*
- *Can be localized. When found in an isolated area only (not affecting both eyes) it is an IRRITANT.*

ALLERGIC DERMATITIS- *can develop over time of wearing extensions. Other factors also come into play: Body chemistry changes, immune deficiency, stress, and other diseases, and skin conditions are a huge factor.*

Seasonal Allergies- *switching to a sensitive adhesive for periods at a time is an alternative. Or suggest a break for the eyes to rest.*

TRACTION ALOPECIA

Repeated use of eyelash extensions can cause traction alopecia, a condition where the hair falls out due to excessive tension placed on the hair shaft. Damage to the hair follicle is irreversible, slowing down to ceasing growth of the hair. Using the incorrect size, diameters and lack of separation in the procedure are causes of traction alopecia.

OCULAR ROSACEA

Condition associated with rosacea in general. It is an inflammatory skin condition. Rosacea is triggered by different factors and usually shows signs of redness on the cheeks, nose and neck. Broken blood vessels and acne like bumps may be present in around the eye area or very close. If signs are present on the clients face, there is a likely chance he/she will have ocular rosacea. Remember that all people are chemically different and some react far less or far more than others.

For some individuals rosacea is not present and may be present in the eye area after an application (or several) to come to surface. Usually affect mid-aged individuals. No cure is available for this condition. Medical advice or a dermatologist opinion is recommended for clients who have questions outside the scope of practice. (Remember: diagnosing is not in the scope of practice)

CANCER

Is it a good idea to provide lash extensions on a client? I can honestly say that if you're an experience artist you can make an educated decision on when it is ok to service a client. It is always best to be conservative on the application, choosing a thin diameter and realistic sizes that mimic the natural lash length. Each client has a different experience for hair loss during cancer treatment. Some may lose all their lashes while others do not. A client typically will demand length and drama to compensate out of fear of what is to come. The self-appearance and self-care is important to the client. You must remember your goal is the natural state of the lash and health. Be firm and educate the client on safety. The skin suffers tremendously and changes during treatment and sensitivities occur. It is wiser to wait until treatment is nearing the end and signs of hair growth is in sight. Make note your clients body is still purging the chemicals from treatment and trying to breed the 'healthy' flora. So though signs of hair growth is coming in; it can and will not grow to full potential for sometime. It begins then seizes growth because of the toxins still being purged through the skin. It does take months after the last treatment for the client to recover in skin conditions and hair growth.

CHAPTER FOUR

PROTOCOLS

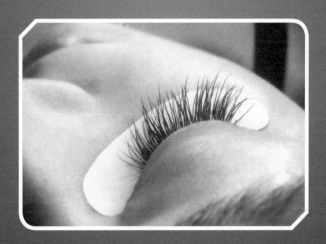

PREP- PROCEDURE PROTOCOL
PREPARING FOR YOUR WORK ENVIRONMENT

Equipment is key -> keep it simple.
- Invest in a table that is comfortable for you. A massage table works great as long as you can get your legs under so you can practice proper posture. An esthetician table that can rotate with hydraulics is best. Clients vary in height and size so you may have to adjust your station for different clients.
- Mag-lamp\ professional lighting for procedures is a must.
- Store your products in a case if possible.
- Practice proper sanitation for your tools (remember you are working in the eye region a delicate area)
- Use of gloves on both hands a must. Bacteria, dirt, and oils are on the skin. You may have dirt stuck in your nails. The membrane of the eye area is delicate. It does not take much to irritate the eye.
- Design a consent form to legally protect you and the business.
- Get in the practice of keeping soap (clinical) notes on your sessions recording any changes to your work, client comments, etc.

POSTURE & MOBILITY
Comfort is important. BE comfortable first. Then your client's comfort comes next. If you don't have proper posture your work will be unsatisfactory. You are stationary for long periods of time, which could lead to posture health issue. Keep your core strong and engaged. The head of the client should be at chest level to you. Rotational tables or fixed treatment tables work fine. In my opinion, as a practitioner, I prefer a table that has hydraulics for movement.

Tips - Suggestions

- Prepare your treatment table with proper draping paper.
- Your station should be clean and clutter free. Remember that promoting a clean working space gives the client confidence that you have best practices in place for sanitation and cleanliness.
- Wash your hands and have clean tools properly wrapped in a sanitation pouch.
- Before starting the cleansing process, make sure your chair is in proper height and you have comfortable access to the face and a bird's eye view of the eyes.

LASH EXTENSION PROCEDURE PROTOCOL
Pre-Cleanse Procedure

Cleanse the eye area. Remove any makeup and mascara. A gentle eyewash or a sensitive face cleanser can also be used. I suggest a product that will strip the oil from the natural lash. Many professional artists would agree that baby shampoo is a great product to use.

Gel Patch Application: Place one patch on the eye. Make sure the patch is 1-2 millimeters away from the waterline base of bottom lid. You should be able to see the base of the bottom lash. The gel patch should not push up into the eye. Have the client close her eye before sealing the patch in place. Have her hold lightly the eye gel patch in place; while you place the second patch on the other eye. Holding the first patch in place and aiding the lid keeps it from opening while working on the other eye. If the client opens her eyes, the patch can/will shift up creating potential discomfort. Check each eye once more to make sure bottom lashes are secure or if a re-adjustment needs to be done.

Gloves. Put gloves on after gel patch placement. Gloves will stick to the gel patch in most cases making it difficult to get the gel patch aligned correctly.

Use a mascara brush to comb through the lashes. Try to direct them in a straight direction. Brushing lashes will also help any Telogen lashes on the verge of shedding to possibly release.

Analysis of the eyes and make note of what you notice.
- Does the client have any gaps in certain areas?
- Take notice of where her longest lashes are located.
- Are her corners short or sparse?
- Thin versus thick diameter?
- Is the lid skin loose?
- Skin dry? Any signs of allergies present?
- Is the lids pink or skin color pigment?
- Do you notice anything else that may be important to address or note?

Cleansing the eye area is important for the following reasons:
Removal of makeup, dust, oil and mucous buildup gives you a clean pallet of natural lashes to work with. Oil builds up around the cuticle of the natural lash. If excess oil is not removed, proper absorption of the adhesive will be prevented. The oil causes a barrier between the natural lash and the extension from fusing together 100%. If spaces, air pockets or slip occurs, the lashes will fall prematurely (not lasting as long as it should).

Adhering extensions to lashes that are dirty is not proper hygienic practice. Mites or other discomfort to the client and other eye irritant issues can arise.

Use makeup remover, cleanser and cleansing technique to prepare your client at each lash service. Never skip the cleansing protocol.

Use a mascara brush to remove debris that pack around the base of the lid and natural hair.

ADHESIVE: CHEMICAL AGENTS

Information about different adhesives depends on the distributor or manufacturer that the lash artist is purchasing from. There are several companies in the market that sell adhesive appropriate for different practitioners and location. The climate along with humidity in the workspace plays a factor on the success of the bonding agent. Bonding Agents can vary with regards to resistant to water and oils. Companies can provide specific instructions on proper use of the adhesives and storage. It is important to request the material safety data sheet (MSDS) info for a copy for your product records in your business. MSDS provides a summary of the product and valuable information in case an incident occurs with a client. Each adhesive may have instructions on how to use it correctly and get the most mileage out of your bond. Some require primer preparation before using the adhesive; others do not. Humidity in the atmosphere or chemicals that harness and deplete the moisture in the air can interfere with chemical structure of the bonding agent. An example of products that counteract would be hair color mixtures or strong hair setting services like the Brazilian hair straighteners. Running a humidifier or maintaining a controlled air environment should be considered. Heating and Air conditioning units can also deplete the moisture in your workspace. Tip: Keep a Nano Mister on hand for the service. The mist accelerates the activation of the molecules in the adhesive to compress together going from a liquid to a solid form.

GENERAL INFORMATION : ADHESIVE.

The base ingredient in adhesive is *cyanoacrylate.* There are different chemical cyanoacrylates used for cosmetic and industrial purposes. The base is a resin that polymerizes when in contact with moisture. Those sensitive to acrylics risk a chance of a reaction to the adhesive. A small pin sized amount of adhesive is all that is needed for application.

Medical Grade: Octyl & Butyl Cyanoacrylate - Used in surgical procedures and types of wound closures.

Industrial Mainly: Methyl & Ethyl Cyanoacrylate - Popular because it is quick drying

PRIMERS & SEALANTS

The primer strips the lash to prepare the suction process of the bond. * Primers have been reported of contributing towards reactions. The adhesives bonding compound should be enough for application. A lash artist might chose to use a sealant after curing the lashes as the final step of the procedure. Waiting 12 - 24 hours before exposure to getting immersed in water is recommended for the longevity of retention.

NANO- Mister: I highly recommend misting! It aids in eliminating the vapors of the fume and cures that bonding faster than just air alone. It removes the stinging sensation a client may experience.

APPLICATION TOOLS

You will need 2 different shaped tweezers; straight tweezers for application and a curved tweezers for isolation. For volume you will need a curved or flat tip tweezers instead of a straight tweezers. Hand and wrist control is essential during application. How you hold your tools and proper hand positioning will decrease future potential problems of arm and hand fatigue and possible carpal tunnel syndrome. Please take this seriously for the longevity of your career. Avoid placing too much pressure in the fingers while holding the isolation tweezers...this prevents pressure on the lower pads and lids. Maintain a sturdy grip without stressing the hands and fingers. Prevent fatigue on the muscles of the phalanges, wrist and joints. Stretch your hands often.

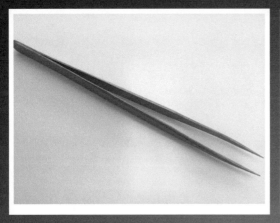
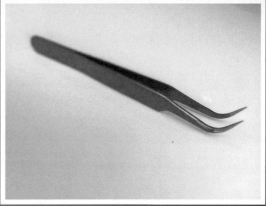

GENERAL PROTOCOLS
LASH PICKUP/ ISOLATION PROTOCOL - Hands On Practice
Select and prepare the extension dipping into the adhesive first. Then go in to separate/ isolate... then place the extension. Preparing the extension first is safest, allowing your eye to stay on the target of application.

*Separation before picking up the lash when you are a beginner is not recommended.

SEPARATION OF THE LASHES PROTOCOL
Separation of the dry extensions from neighboring extensions and natural lashes must be performed and is extremely important. If it is not done correctly, the client will feel like she has a clumped section of lashes causing a sensation of pinprick. A pinprick is a hypersensitive pinch reaction that can lead a client to picking and pulling leading to increase potential lash damage. This is a sign that a lash is causing a disturbance. Working from one eye to the next in a back and forth routine; between rounds do a separation. Separation will allow the extensions to fluff up. The final result looks fuller. An additional benefit is the ability to find natural lashes that may have been missed during the application process.

When separating with the isolation and application tweezers, it is important for one hand to remain stable while the other does the peeling and pulling away.

REMOVAL METHODS

There are 2 methods.

1. Micro-brush / Liquid Removal Method

Stroke each lash with the brush about 2-4 times. Allow the removal to set for 7-10 minutes. The adhesive will liquefy from the solid form. The lash will slip off one by one.

2. Peeling Method (banana peel)

There are several ways to perform this removal. Depending on the hair you are trying to remove, the movement must be done slowly and with sturdy control of the wrist and hands. The lash extension can be bent slightly at the base causing it to lift. Use one of the tweezers to keep the natural lash in place and the other tweezers to peel away. Or, if the hair splits along the pre-tapered tip, start from the top and peel back gently while stabilizing the natural hair in place. Always stabilize the natural lash in place to avoid pulling/plucking out. If peeled incorrectly, the natural hair will curl such as a pair of scissors dragging a straight ribbon to get it to curl when decorating a gift box. The peeling method is best used to remove a stubborn lash during the lash fill clean up protocol before you begin a fill. Or when a client wants a removal of the very little lash extensions she may have left from several weeks of application.

TOUCH UP

Your client loved her lashes; now the time has arrived for her lash fill. The touch up is a whole different game. It's not a full set but it's another learning curve ball. This course is important to teach you (the artist) all the different aspects of applying lash extensions and the dedication it takes to be a great *LASH SPECIALIST*. The aim is to teach you this exceptional career from the start and the continuation of keeping your clients loyal.

The touch up process can be a bit frustrating versus starting from the beginning. Remember that at least 15-20% of the clients remaining lashes will have to be removed. The reasons are following:

1. Dislodged extension must be removed no matter what! The lifting at the base of the extension can cause puckering during blinking leading to an irritated lid in a particular section of the eye. In most cases a client does not feel it. But clients do notice the growth between the base extension and the lid.
2. If the natural lash has grown into the second or third stage, the growth that isn't supported by the base of the lash will cause the lash to sway over side ways or almost appear upside down becoming an irritant if not resized at the time of appointment.
3. Lash Extensions that are not resized will look unattractive; giving the illusion that the client is in need of a fill.
4. Lashes that are long and flopping could be that either the extensions were to long to begin with for the natural lash. OR not enough shorter lash extensions applied to the original look. Short lash extensions are important to support the long extensions creating a frame of support. * Refer back to pg. 4 the discussion of "Building a House".
5. Most importantly, don't forget to wash / cleanse the lashes before you get started!!!

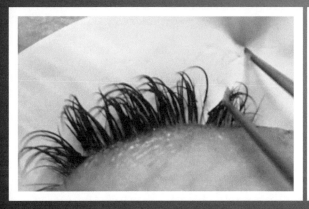 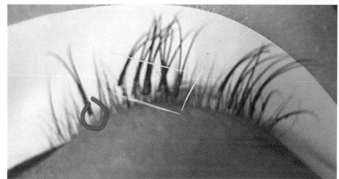

ALLERGIC IRRITANT REACTION PROTOCOL

Your client has a reaction; what now? It can be very uncomfortable for new lash specialist to feel a bit nervous when a client's eyes show signs of a reaction. Envision yourself in your client's shoes. Immediately follow up with your client. Do not hesitate or ignore her and down play the reaction. Insist for her to come in so that you can do an assessment and proceed with further action. These could be a possible removal and/or direct medical attention. Remember stay within the scope of your practice.

Tips / Suggestions
To avoid any potential communication problems, always make sure you have a client fill out a company consent form prior to her initial visit. It is VERY IMPORTANT the client understands the procedure and signs the proper forms in your practice. Do not miss even a date. The form is not valid if it is not 100% complete.

Once the reaction has been reported, ask the client to come in so that you can evaluate the severity of the reaction. Clients can sometimes under or over explain the severity. Make no suggestions until you see her in person or have her email you immediately pictures of her reaction for your records. Irritant: check to make sure that an individual lash is not dislodged. Check the distance of the lash to the lash line… is it to close?

Depending on the severity, lash removal may be necessary.

When sending a client to seek medical evaluation, fill out an incident report and attach it to the consent form.

Some thoughts or questions to consider: If a client has had lashes prior at a different location, ask her if she ever had any signs of a minor indication. This can happen and the client did not feel that it was significant to mention it or just not on her mind. But then the reaction occurs and the concerns begin.

Some clients have a irritant sensitivity much like a seasonal allergy and an antihistamine has been known to help. A client may take it prior to a visit and helps lessen the severity. Though it is best to make the right decision and turn down the service when appropriate.

You are not a doctor. It is outside of your scope of practice to prescribe any medication or ointment. Do NOT diagnose any ocular disease or disorder. Have her seek medical advice or consent prior to her lash procedure.

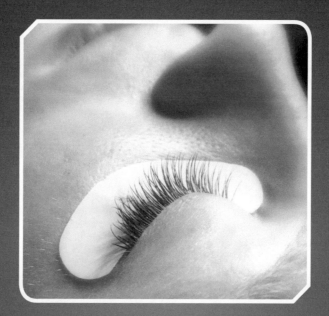

EYE PATCHES
SEALING THE LOWER LASHES

Finding the right patches that feel the most comfortable for the client is important. Below are some different methods. The favorable method is gel patches. Medical Tape is a NO. You will see several artists showcase their work on social media with medical tape.

*In class discussion about the proper use of medical tape will go into more detail about best use.

Gel Patches come in different shapes. The gel substance varies from manufacturer and vendor. We offer a few different options for you to try and see what works best for you. It's important to know that with the many selections of gel patches, the gel substance can be packed with chemicals that can cause a reaction.

Eye Stickers aid in the stability of various gel patches when you use them together. But you can also use them alone. Some stickers are thinner than others.

*Be careful when using them. Can cause corneal abrasions due to the rounded edges. Paper cuts hurt – stickers can do that to the conjunctiva.

Medical Tape - huge NO! Medical tape is harsh on the skin and to the natural bottom lashes. It also looks very unprofessional. Medical Tape is a tool to use to aid an application for the beginner.

Silicone Eye Pads are hypoallergenic and reusable. Just another option for the lash specialist that may like them.

Avoid using medical tape as a substitute for gel patches or eye stickers. Medical tape is harsh for the delicate under eye.

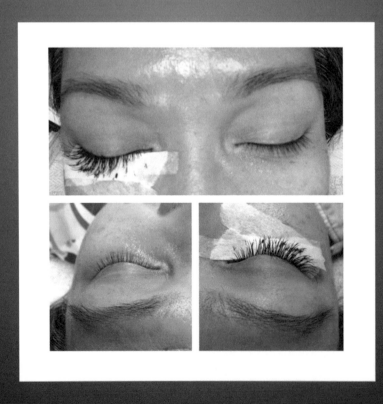

CHAPTER FIVE

EMPOWERING & CUSTOMIZE

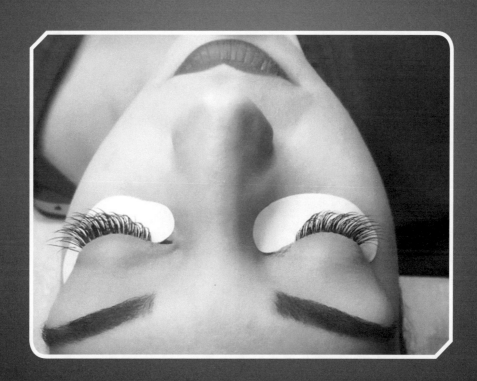

ART OF FRAMING

Placement is an art. The advantage is the stage of the hair will guide you on what is the appropriate size for placement. If you follow the health and safety of placement to maintain the integrity of the natural lash, then most of the framing is done.

FACE FACTORS

Look at the entire big picture (face)
- What is the focal point feature of the face?
- What physical feature needs to be enhanced or down played?
- What is the natural shape of the eye?
- Symmetry of the eyes
- Brows! Look at the arch. Is the arch defined? Where is the high point?
- Can you alter the shape/ enhance differently?
- What is the expectation of the client?
- Is the expectation realistic?
- How does the client define natural versus dramatic?
- What your clients needs?
- Do her eyes need to appear bigger or smaller?
- Any obvious signs of prior lash damage?
- Gaps in her lashes?

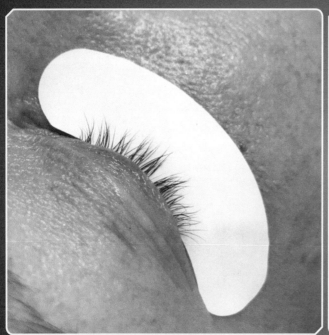
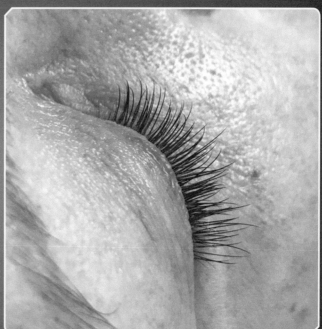

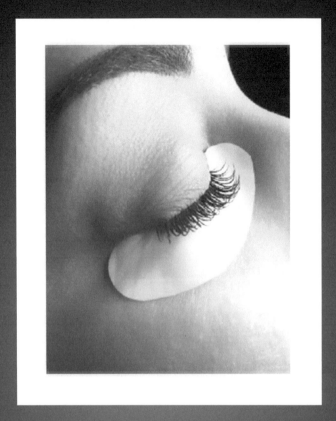

FACE SHAPE TIPS

The client's eye shape is the foundation of the customized look you will create. The following are tips to guide you on your selection of sizes you will use. The lash map provided in the business kit is a great cheat sheet for a beginner practitioner.

DIFFERENT EYE SHAPES

1. **Close Set Eyes**: Tip Flare outer corners make it denser (thicker) sparingly towards inner corner (the objective here is the flare makes the statement taking away from the illusion of the eyes set to close to each other.

2. **Monolid Eyes** (Common mostly in Asian): NO crease just a single eyelid. Shapes such as B Shape plane the base of the straight lash up to give it a curl. Asians

usually have straight no curve lashes. Another option depending on the length of the lash; L shape works great and gives the illusion of a lid. Place the longest sizes on the lashes located in the center of the eyelid. It makes the eye structure appear open.

3. **Hooded Eyes** (droopy skin): The crease is hidden the best lashes to use C curl or D curl. Lifts the eye open -hiding the droopy skin.

4. **Protruding Eyes** (bulging appearance): B shape and doing a few 12's mostly 10's and 9's frame the eye to reduce the bulging.

5. **Upward Eyes** - The outer corners have a natural lift and the inner part goes downward. Most clients want to accentuate the cat eye. Don't. Use smaller extensions in the corner and towards the center mid section use longer lashes sparingly. You don't want their eyes to look smaller.

6. **Downward Eyes** – Downward in the outer corner- avoid cat eye! Avoid putting lashes in the far corners and start a quarter in with lashes to give the illusion of a length.

7. **Almond Shape** – a common balanced shape. Creativity using the Face Factors to design a look.

LASH MAPPING
MANNEQUIN HANDS-ON

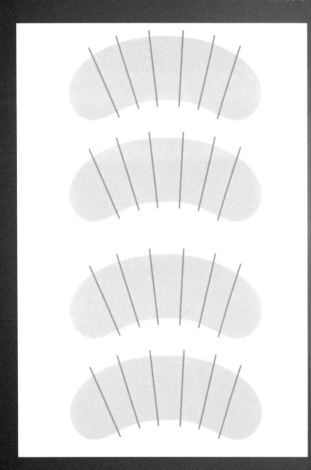

Lash mapping is a great tool for a lash specialist who is learning. The lines on a lash map sticker allow you to pen in the sizes to guide the customized look.

CHAPTER SIX

GENERAL PROTOCOLS

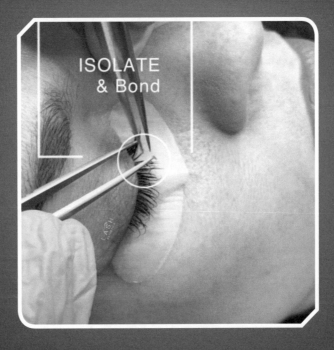

"BE LASHED... BE BOLD"

JESSICA GONZALEZ

AFTERCARE PROTOCOL + PRODUCTS

- ***Cleaners & Cleansing Brush***: Include an aftercare guideline for the client. Lash Extensions is an investment. Think about offering a gift with service for the first time client. Putting together a selection of must have products for the client and having it ready for purchase makes it easy for the client to be informed on what to use. And avoids exposure to other products she may feel tempted to use that could potentially break down the lash extensions sooner.
- **Mascara**: The truth is lash extensions make a HUGE difference to the appearance. Powerful than what can be achieved alone. But many clients will want more than less at least 60% of the time. Stock up on lash extensions friendly mascara at the register. Thus your client doesn't have to go sneaking around about using mascara for the in-between fill visits. (Waterproof mascara is a sin)
- **Mascara WAND brushing:** Brushing is great for the lashes! It keeps them straight and untangled. But a heavy hand must be avoided. Lashes need a tender touch to the brush! Demonstrate on the client and give them a brush to take home with them.
- **Lash Lock Sealer (s)** – a must have for clients who may loose lashes faster than normal. Or have active lifestyles evolving body sweat for example. Using this product every couple of days seals in the lash when it starts to dislodge from the natural lash. Clients who travel a lot, love to have this product on hand.
- **Lash Serum Advantage** – Encourage clients to use a serum. With consistence they work fabulously and keep the natural lash nourished. Many serums are commonly available in the market.

*This manual is to provide general information without being focused on brands of products. Ask your instructor during class what her favorite products are that she may suggest

PRICING YOUR SERVICE WITH CONFIDENCE

Demographics, location, niche, and value in your education must be considered when determining your value of services. Get paid what your worth. With knowledge comes power and confidence. Stand your ground on standards regardless of other service providers in your area. How much is your time worth? When the suggested price is higher in price, it allows you the leverage to run promotions and still have lucrative success.

General Price Suggestions
Classic full set suggested pricing $100-$150 for an independent service provider, and a spa/salon should charge $150-200 or higher. Location, demographics, product selection, and expertise are factors when considering the price for the menu.

Hybrid or volume full sets pricing average is $200-300. Consider the time invested, product cost, and the assessment of the clients natural lashes. It can take up to 2 -3 hours for this particular application technique.

Lash Touch Ups (Increase $10-20 more for enhancements in hybrid or volume)
- 2 Week: $50-65
- 3 week: $65-75
- 4 week: $75-85
- 5 weeks $100 and up.

Removal can be complimentary for existing clients. Walk in non-clients service cost is estimated at $45. Apply the removal fee as a discount when a client comes in for a lash service in the future. An unhappy client from a different location can be a loyal client opportunity if you seize the moment to educate her on the art of lash extensions.

POLICY & FORMS
INSURANCE
Obtaining additional insurance or adding the service to your current policy varies in each state. Research your state for regulations. Independent contractors must be self-insured. As a business owner with employees the business should have each practitioner insured. Liability Insurance is a must.

- *Marine Agency offers insurance*
- *ASCP offers liability insurance*

FORMS

A general consent form for the service is a must. Consult with your advisors/lawyers regarding the specific structure of business and structure of your forms.

Suggested Documents For Business Record Keeping
- Consent Health Form
- Company Refund Policy Form
- Lash Log Form
- Removal Form
- Incident Form

THE CONSULT PROCEDURE

Review the forms, ask important questions and address the expectations of the client. This is a review of the Chapter 5 "Art Of Framing".

Some questions to ask:
1. *Have you had any prior experience with eyelash extensions? If so, tell me what you did or didn't like.*
2. *How many layers of mascara are you accustom to applying?*
3. *Do you like the length you have when you do wear mascara?*
4. *Do you use a curler? (This gives you an idea of what shape you may want to use)*
5. *Any regular or seasonal allergies?*
6. *What are your symptoms? Knowing what the effects of the allergies helps determining the size or diameter that may work best to reduce or avoid any potential irritants.*

7. *Look at your client's features. The size of her eyes, and significant features. Do you want to highlight the shape of eye? Are the eyes smaller and need to appear wider and give a slightly bigger illusion?*

Charging for consultations
YES! I highly recommend to keep your fee at a modest price of $25-50. Offer to apply the consult charge towards the cost of the full set service if the client books with you.

SANITATION | HYGIENE PRACTICES
Follow your state regulations.
1. Sanitize your tools immediately with an approved proper agent.
2. Store tools in a sealed pouch.
3. Use Disposable mascara / micro brushes / glue rings (change with each client)
4. Sanitize your treatment table after each client with approved medical grade solution.
5. Wash hands at start of service
6. Make sure all consent forms are properly and completely filled and signed.
7. Keep a sanitation log if your town / state requires it. It is a best practice and it covers your steps!

MARKETING
- Do you have an established business?
- Describe the business demographics (client profile)
- Who is the Ideal client?
- Plan of action of introduction of your new service
- Menu and business cards
- Network with local business in your area
- Use of social networks. It is important to choose one or two at the most that will be the most effective. Do not overwhelm yourself with the use of to many platforms. Chose the one and maximize on your content.

- Set the price based on the target market and area analysis. Be realistic. Though do not sell yourself short on your talents.
- BE CONFIDENT
- BE KNOWLEDABLE. Educate your clients. Encourage and welcome questions.
- Network with other professionals.

Are you ready to grow your lash career? I hope this manual provided a great introductory in your new journey. The information in this manual is for informational and educational purposes. Use as a guide to reference in your lash practice. Stay fresh, stay focused and become the best lash specialist you can be. Wishing you a career of lashing with passion as much as I have!

Light & Grace,

Jessica Gonzalez

Printed in the United States
By Bookmasters